Lose a stone in six weeks!

the Booster Plan!

Contents

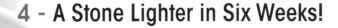

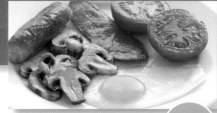

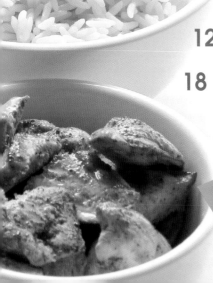

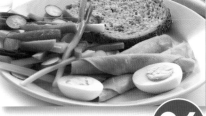

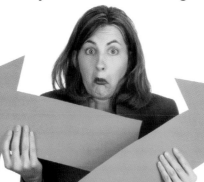

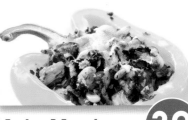

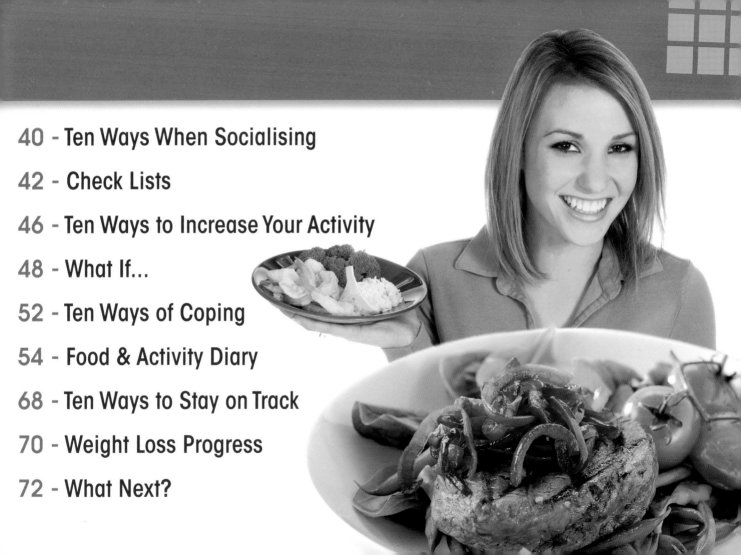

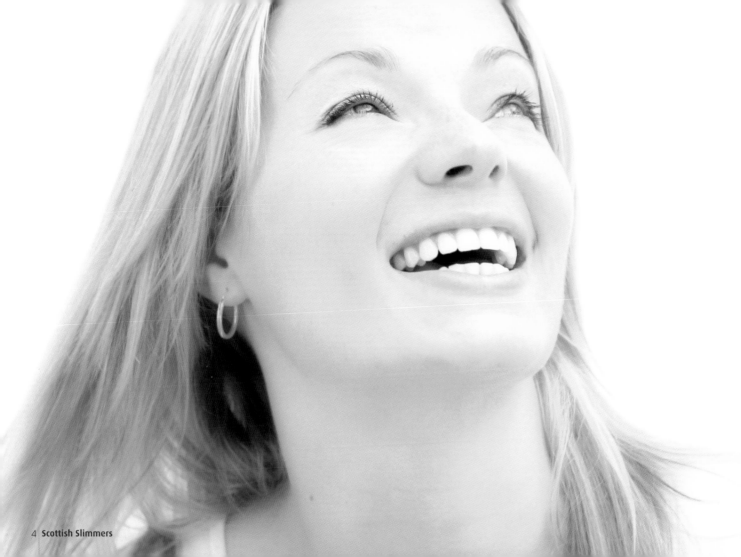

A stone lighter
in six weeks!

Losing one stone can make an enormous difference to the way you look and feel!

It's a great psychological milestone and, for most women, it will mean dropping at least one dress size – possibly two.

Make no bones about it, losing one stone is a tremendous achievement. We often forget that – especially if our intention is to lose several stones – but ask anyone who has lost several stones how they felt as each stone dropped off and many will tell you that it was focussing on just one stone at a time that enabled them to reach their ultimate goal.

Generally speaking, most people can comfortably lose 1-2lb a week following a healthy weight loss plan such as the Positive Eating Plan.

To lose 14lb in six weeks means you really will need to pull out all the stops!

It's also true to say that all stones are not equal – as you get lighter each stone is a little more challenging and may take longer to lose than when you were heavier, or just starting on a weight loss plan.

We've prepared a special plan in this book which, if followed for six weeks, should give you your best possible result. We've no intention of starving you, nor insisting you spend three hours a day down the gym, but, if you are prepared to give it all you've got, this slightly different approach to Positive Eating is just what you need!

Ten Ways to
Get Motivated

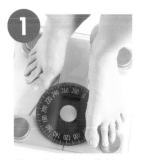

1

Aim to be 1 stone lighter in six weeks time (or at least aim to lose more weight than you lost in the last six weeks).

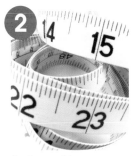

2

Aim for a waist measurement that's 5 cm/2 inches smaller in six weeks' time.

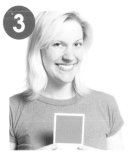

3

Sort out a photo of yourself at a weight you liked.

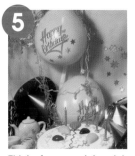

4

Find an item of clothing in your wardrobe about one or two sizes too small that you'd really like to get back into.

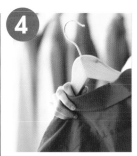

5

Think of any special social occasion you might have to attend in about six weeks' time.

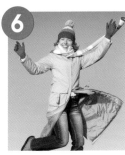

6

Keep remembering that losing 1 stone will make it easier to walk and run, and will help lower blood pressure, lower cholesterol levels and improve blood sugar levels.

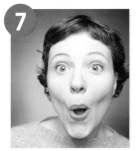

7

Think about who'll be impressed!

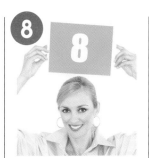

8

At the end of each day, award yourself a mental mark out of ten – depending on how well you've kept to your eating and activity plan (or jot it down on your food diary).

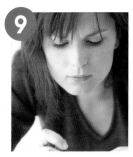

9

Set a six week period and stick to this plan as closely as you can, on every day that you can. If you don't manage every single day, don't feel you have to keep starting again at the beginning. Just keep going for six weeks and see what you can achieve.

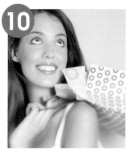

10

Plan a reward for your achievement.

How do I get started?

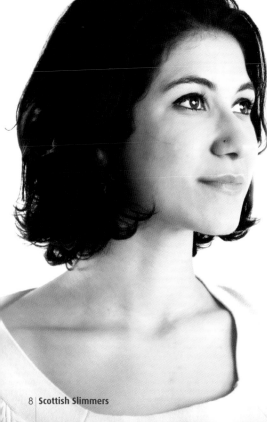

You can follow this plan in much the same way as any other Positive Eating Plan – **but there is one major difference.**

On this plan, there are more foods that don't need to be counted such as lean meat, fish, Quorn, pulses, low-fat milks, low-fat cheeses, yoghurt and fromage frais. (You can find a full list of these "No-Need-To-Count" foods on page 12.)

For other items, women have a daily allowance of 20 Checks and men 30 Checks.

In addition, you have a Special Weekly Allowance of an extra 20 Checks to spend if you want. This means you don't have to "save" from your daily Checks allowance for special weekend treats, etc.

You should still also have your Every Day Bonus foods as on all Positive Eating Plans. (There is a reminder of these on page 10.)

TO SUMMARISE, THIS IS WHAT YOU SHOULD HAVE EACH DAY:

Every Day Bonus foods
(not forgetting free drinks, free vegetables, free additions)

No-Need-To-Count foods.

20 Checks a day to spend as you please on other items
(or 30 Checks if you are a man).

A Special Weekly Allowance of 20 Checks to spend if you want.

You can either make up your own meals and snacks, using No-Need-To-Count foods, Every Day Bonus foods and adding other items using your daily Checks allowance.

Or, you can use the meal ideas in this book which tell you how many Checks you need to count from your daily allowance of 20 Checks (30 for men). Any remaining Checks may be spent as you please, and don't forget to have your Every Day Bonus foods also.

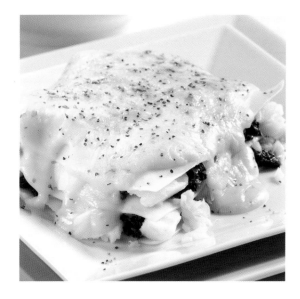

Every Day Bonus

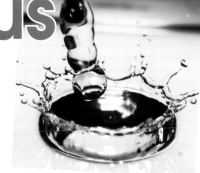

Every Day Bonus foods are included in all Positive Eating Plans. Try to have them every day as they provide many essential nutrients for good health. Here is a reminder of them, but you can find full details in your Positive Eating Plan. You don't have to spend any Checks on these daily allowances and No-Check foods.

Liquid Assets

Each day have at least 8 cups/glasses of fluid. Water, tea, coffee and low-calorie "diet" drinks that contain 3 or fewer calories per 100ml may be drunk freely.

Bone Builders

These foods are high in calcium to build and maintain strong bones. Choose one item a day from the following, or have half of one and half of another. On this plan the quantities given are the minimum you need each day, but as the following are also No-Need-To-Count foods, you can have more if you wish.

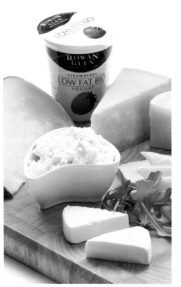

- *275ml skimmed milk*
- *200g pot or 2 x 125g pots virtually-fat-free natural or flavoured yoghurt*
- *200g virtually-fat-free natural or flavoured fromage frais*
- *150g pot 0% fat natural Greek yoghurt.*
- *40g half-fat cheese*
- *50g low-fat/light soft cheese*
- *75g extra light soft cheese*
- *100g quark or cottage cheese*

See page 16 for other No-Need-To-Count dairy foods.

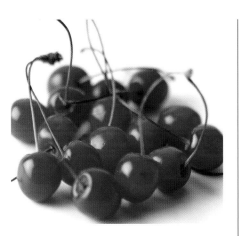

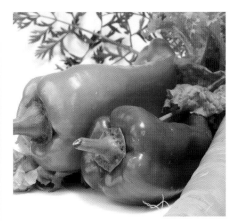

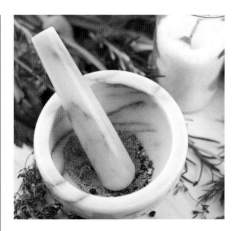

Fruit

Have 2 "average" servings of fruit each day. An average serving is a medium round fruit such as an apple, orange, peach or pear. Or, 2 small fruits such as satsumas, figs, small kiwi fruits. Or, 85g grapes. Or, 225g berries. Or 300g with skin/200g peeled melon. Or, 100g canned fruit in juice. Or, 100ml unsweetened fruit juice.

The following fruits count as 2 servings – a large cooking apple, a medium banana, a medium mango or papaya.

Vegetables

The following vegetables may be eaten freely, but aim to have at least 3 servings each day so that together with your 2 servings of fruit you will be having your 5-a-day.

artichokes, asparagus, aubergine, baby sweetcorn, beansprouts, beetroot, broccoli, brussels sprouts, cabbage, carrots, cauliflower, celery, courgettes, cress, cucumber, fennel, green beans, greens, leeks, lettuce, mangetout, marrow, mushrooms, onions, peppers, pumpkin, radishes, spinach, swede, tomatoes, turnips, watercress

Free additions

Many foods used for taste and flavour are used in very small quantities and have negligible calories so don't need to be counted. These include:

artificial sweeteners, Bovril, egg white, essences/extracts, gelatine, herbs, Marmite, rhubarb, spices, stock cubes/granules, tomato purée, spices, spray oil, sugar-free gum, sugar-free jelly, salt, pepper, mustard, vinegar, lemon/lime juice, mint sauce, pickled vegetables, soy sauce, Tabasco/chilli sauce, Worcestershire sauce.

See Every Day Bonus section of your Positive Eating Plan for full details.

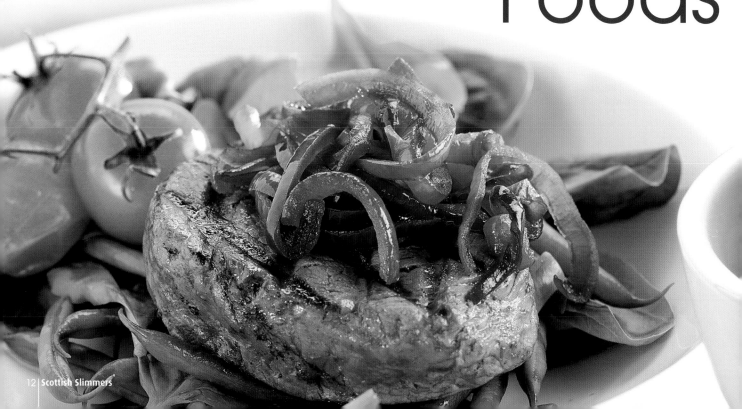

No-Need-To-Count
Foods

This plan is different from all our other Positive Eating Plans.

Your daily Checks allowance is lower than usual – because there are lots more foods on this plan that you don't have to count and which may be eaten freely according to your appetite.

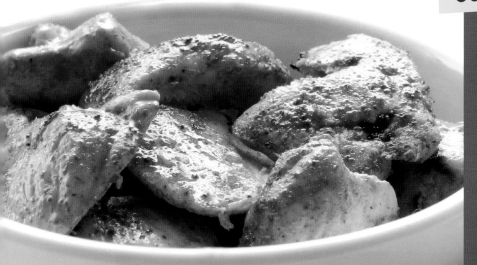

Use common sense!

Whilst you don't have to count these foods from your Checks allowance, try not to have excessively large portions of No-Need-To-Count foods, or you could find your weight loss slows down.

Meat

Any lean, fat-trimmed, skinless meat including:

Beef

Chicken

Duck

Game birds

Kidney *

Lamb

Liver *

Mince, any up to10% fat

Pork

Rabbit

Turkey

Venison

Back bacon

Bacon medallions

Turkey rashers

Bresaola

Corned beef

Ham

Pastrami

Proscuitto

Wall's Lean Recipe sausages, or similar very low-fat sausages up to 75 calories each.

* Best avoided by women of child-bearing age.

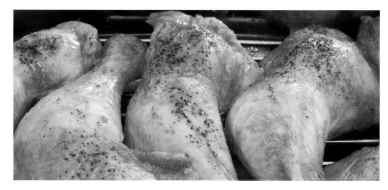

Any "healthy eating" prepared meat dish such as the following, but restrict to one medium portion per day:

Asda Good For You! Mango & Ginger Chicken

Asda Good For You! Pork Steak with a Three Mustard Sauce

Marks & Spencer Count On Us Braised Steak

Marks & Spencer Count On Us Chicken Forestière

Sainsbury's Be Good To Yourself Beef & Red Wine Casserole

Sainsbury's Be Good To Yourself Lamb & Rosemary Casserole

Tesco Healthy Living Chicken Breast in Creamy Mushroom Sauce

Tesco Healthy Living Chicken Breast in Tomato & Basil Sauce

Iceland Good Choice Quarter Pounder

Tesco Healthy Living Quarter Pounder

Or, similar products.

Fish

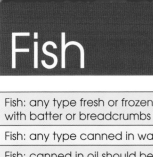

Fish: any type fresh or frozen as long as it is not coated with batter or breadcrumbs
Fish: any type canned in water, brine or tomato sauce
Fish: canned in oil should be well drained
Crustaceans: any such as prawns, crab, shrimps, lobster, etc.
Molluscs: any such as mussels, oysters, cockles, whelks, etc.
Seafood sticks
Individual portion frozen fish in parsley or butter sauce.

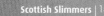

Dairy

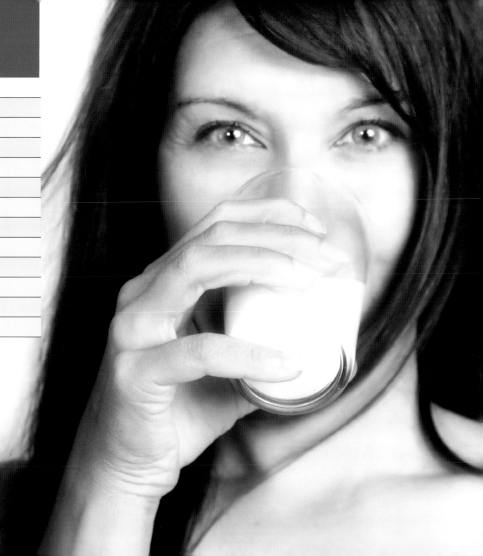

Eggs (up to 7 per week)

Skimmed milk

Virtually-fat-free yoghurt

Virtually-fat-free fromage frais

Cottage cheese

Quark

Half-fat cheese (any type)

Less than 3% fat cheese

Light soft cheese

Extra light soft cheese

Half-fat (light) cheese triangles

Half-fat (light) processed cheese slices

Vegetarian (may also be eaten by non-vegetarians!)

Quorn: mince, pieces, uncoated fillets, balls

Realeat VegeMince or Chicken Style Pieces

Tofu

Soya protein or TVP

Baked beans, preferably reduced-sugar-and-salt

Fresh or frozen peas

Fresh, frozen or canned sweetcorn

Pulses: dried and boiled (e.g. chickpeas, kidney beans, lentils)

Pulses: canned, should be drained and rinsed to remove excess salt

Reduced-fat humous

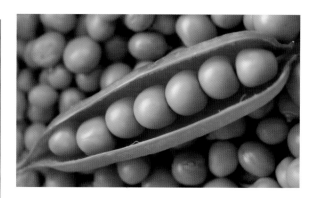

These products also don't need to be counted, but restrict to one medium portion a day (e.g. 2 sausages or burgers).

Cauldren Foods Cumberland Veggie Sausages

Goodlife Organic Vegetable Burgers

Linda McCartney Flame Grilled Burgers

Quorn:
Bangers, Burgers, Chicken Style Roast, Deli Chicken, Ham or Turkey & Stuffing Style Slices, Fajita Strips, Fillets in Tomato & Pepper Sauce, Fillets in White Wine Sauce, Lamb Style Grill, Peppered Steak, Rashers, Sausages (all flavours)

Tivall Burgers or Frankfurters

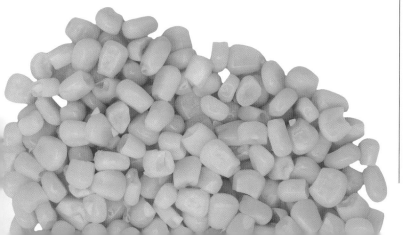

Ten Ways to
Avoid Hunger

1

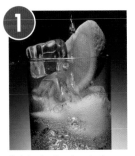

Drink plenty of water/ fluids. Don't mistake thirst for hunger. Avoid excessive amounts of drinks containing caffeine such as coffee, tea and diet cola as these have a diuretic effect.

2

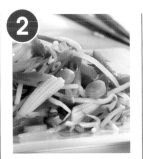

Add lots of No-Check veg to your meals. Steam, stir-fry or microwave for maximum nutrition.

3

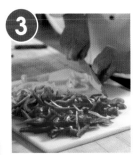

When preparing veg for a meal, peel a few extra to store in the fridge for snacking.

4

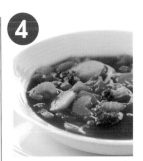

Start a meal with a bowl of soup made from No-Check vegetables, or a bowl of No-Check salad.

5

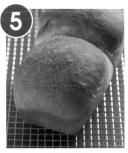

Eat foods high in fibre such as wholemeal or wholegrain breads and cereal, wholemeal pasta and brown rice. The soluble fibre found in oats, apples and pulses is released more slowly and evenly and so helps keep hunger at bay. It can also help lower cholesterol levels.

6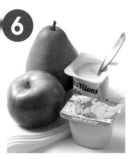

Don't forget your Every Day Bonus foods. Fruit or yoghurt is an ideal between-meal snack.

7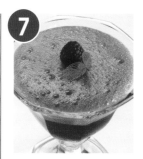

Keep a bowl of sugar-free jelly in the fridge – many of our successful members say it's their lifesaver!

8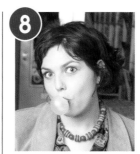

An occasional sugar-free sweet or chewing gum gets you through a sticky moment. Although most sugar-free sweets should be counted, you often get a whole pack for around 4 Checks, which you can spread out over several days.

9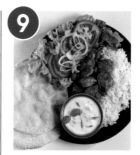

Spread it wide, don't pile it high! The trend for "stacking" food onto a plate gives the impression you're not getting much! Psychologically, a meal seems to be more satisfying if it looks as though you have a full plate, so spread food out (and fill any gaps with No-Check veg).

10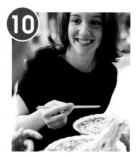

Eat slowly – it takes around 20 minutes for digestive processes to get going and start sending messages to your brain that food is on it's way.

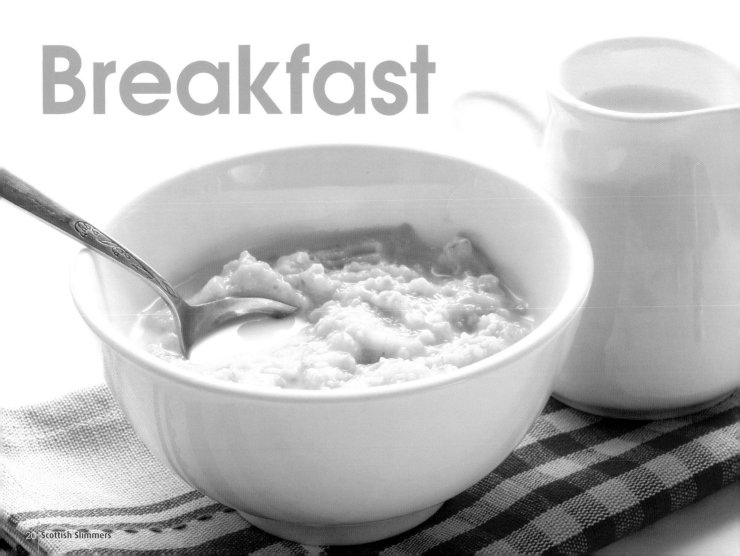

Breakfast

Seriously Simple Checks to count 4

1 sachet Quaker Oatso Simple Original or Ready Brek Seriously Oaty Original, made in the microwave with skimmed milk according to pack instructions. (Checks go up to 6 if you choose a flavoured variety.)

Weetabix Checks to count 5

2 Weetabix with skimmed milk. Add sweetener if required.

Special K Checks to count 4

30g Special K, or Special K Red or Purple Berries, or Special K Peach & Apricot with skimmed milk. Add sweetener if required.

Bran Flakes Checks to count 4

30g bran flakes with skimmed milk. Add sweetener if required.

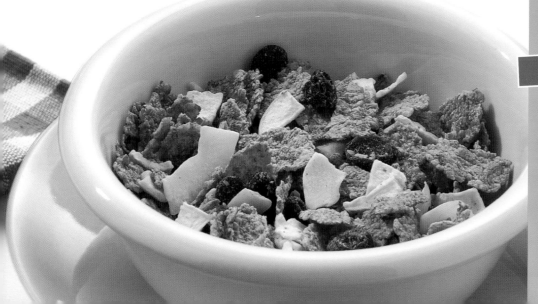

Reminder!

30g of most cereals count as 4 Checks, and you don't need to count anything for skimmed milk or sweetener.

Poached Egg on Smoked Haddock

Poach some smoked haddock in a little skimmed milk and serve topped with a poached egg and grilled tomatoes.

Kipper & Tomatoes

Grill or microwave a kipper or kipper fillets and some tomatoes and serve with 1 medium slice wholemeal bread. (If using "boil-in-the-bag"/microwavable kipper fillets with butter, add 2 Checks).

Smoky Scramble

Scramble an egg with a little skimmed milk. Stir in a few pieces of smoked salmon trimmings and season with black pepper. Serve on 1 medium slice wholemeal toast.

Reminder!

If you wish to add 1 medium slice bread or toast with 1 tsp low-fat spread to any breakfast, you will need to add 4 Checks.

Egg & Ham

Egg(s) poached, dry-fried or scrambled with a little skimmed milk. Serve with lean ham and grilled or microwaved mushrooms.

Rashers, Egg & Waffle

Grill 1 potato waffle, some turkey rashers or bacon medallions and some mushrooms or tomatoes. Serve with egg(s) poached, dry-fried or scrambled with a little skimmed milk.

Sausages & Beans

Grill a couple of very low fat sausages (up to 75 calories each) and serve with baked beans, preferably reduced-sugar-and-salt.

Pan-fried Potatoes & Bacon

Spray a pan with oil and heat. Slice 150g cooked new potatoes, place in the pan and brown on one side, turn over and brown other side. Serve with grilled bacon medallions or turkey rashers and tomatoes or mushrooms.

Egg & Beans

Egg(s) poached, dry-fried or scrambled with a little skimmed milk. Serve with baked beans (preferably reduced-sugar-and salt).

Egg, Sausage & Rasher

Poach or dry-fry 1 egg and serve with 1 grilled very low-fat sausage (up to 75 calories) or 1 Quorn sausage, 1 turkey or Quorn rasher and some mushrooms and tomatoes.

Reminder!

Where a quantity is not given, use your judgement to have as much as you need, but avoid excessively large portions.

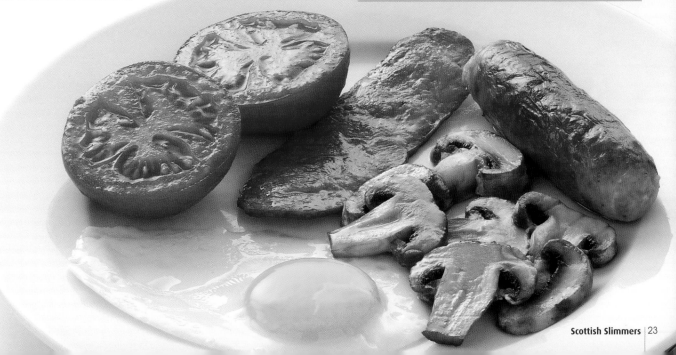

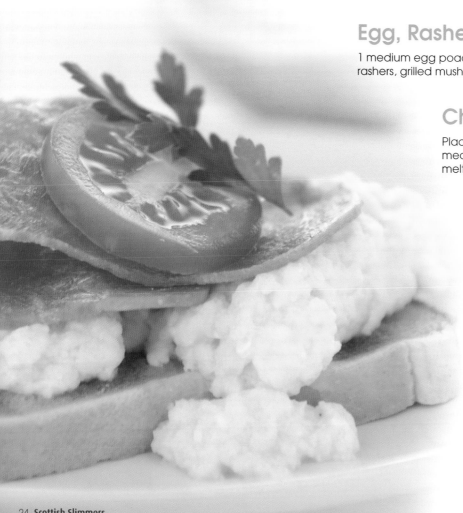

Egg, Rashers & Toast

 Checks to count 3

1 medium egg poached or scrambled, 2 grilled turkey or Quorn rashers, grilled mushrooms or tomatoes, 1 medium slice toast.

Cheese on Toast

 Checks to count 3

Place some sliced or grated half-fat cheddar on 1 medium slice wholemeal toast and grill until cheese melts. Serve with grilled tomatoes.

Boiled/Poached Egg & Toast

Checks to count 3

Boil or poach an egg(s) and serve with 1 medium slice wholemeal toast. Add 1 Check if you wish to spread the toast with low-fat spread.

Toast with Soft Cheese

 Checks to count 3

Top 1 medium slice wholemeal toast with light or extra light soft cheese or cottage cheese.

Microwave Mushroom Omelette

 Checks to count 3

Spray a shallow round dish lightly with oil (e.g. the lid from a Pyrex casserole). Pour in 1 or 2 beaten eggs and some sliced mushrooms. Microwave on high 1-2 minutes. (Timing will depend on microwave power, size of dish, number of eggs and whether or not they have come straight from the fridge.) Serve with 1 medium slice wholemeal bread.

Banana & Yoghurt

 Checks to count 4

1 medium banana and a pot of virtually-fat-free yoghurt (any flavour).

Peach Smoothie

 Checks to count 2

Blitz 1 fresh peach or 2 canned in juice peach halves in a blender together with about 200ml skimmed milk. Add sweetener to taste.

Cereal Bar & Yoghurt

 Checks to count 4

1 Quaker Chewee Bar or Kellogg's Special K Bar or Nestlé Fitnesse Bar, or other bar up to 100 calories, plus a pot of virtually fat free yoghurt (any flavour).

Reminder!

If you use fruit from your Every Day Bonus allowance in your meals, you can deduct 2 Checks for each "average" serving such as an apple, orange or peach. Large pieces of fruit, such as a medium banana or a large cooking apple count as 2 "average" servings, so you can deduct 4 Checks – but remember, once used, you will have to count any other fruit you have during the day.

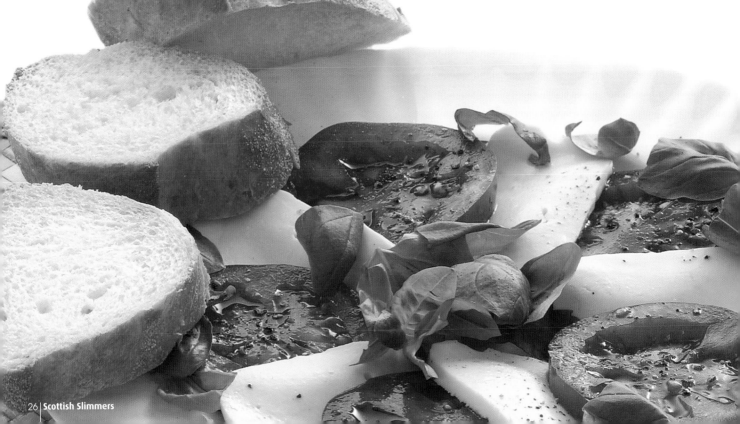

Quick Meals

Mozzarella & Tomato Plate

Slice some half-fat mozzarella and tomatoes and arrange around a plate. Drizzle with oil-free vinaigrette or balsamic vinegar and serve with 3 x 1cm/ ½ inch slices French bread.

Crispbreads with Tuna Topping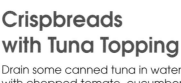

Drain some canned tuna in water or brine and mix with chopped tomato, cucumber, pepper, spring onion. Mix together with either 1 dspn low-calorie mayonnaise or 2 dspn low-calorie salad cream and season with black pepper. Use to top 4 Ryvita Original or Dark Rye crispbreads.

Houmous & Dippers

A medium portion of reduced-fat houmous. Use raw No-Check vegetables such as celery, carrot sticks, chunks of pepper, cauliflower or broccoli florets and 4 breadsticks or Ryvita Original or Dark Rye crispbreads for dipping.

Cheese & Fruit

Serve a medium portion of half-fat cheese with 1 apple and 1 pear.

Spicy Beano

Boil 30g rice or pasta (or use 75g cooked weight) and mix with a can of spicy beans (approx. 200-220g). Serve either warm or cold with additional No-Check salad or vegetables.

Reminder!

Pulses such as beans, chickpeas and lentils are high in soluble fibre, which gives them a low Glycaemic Index rating. Low GI foods release their energy more slowly, so keep you going longer.

Cheese Salad Sandwich

Use 1 tsp low-fat spread to cover 2 medium slices wholemeal bread. Fill with lettuce, tomato and a medium portion of grated half-fat cheese. Add thinly sliced onion or cucumber or other No-Check salad if you wish.

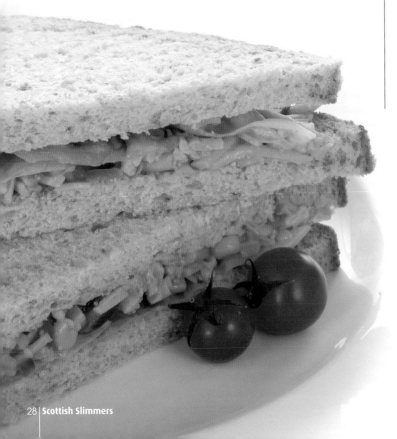

Salmon Sandwich

Drain some canned salmon and mix with chopped cucumber and either 1 dspn low-calorie mayonnaise or 2 dspn low-calorie salad cream. Use to fill 2 medium slices wholemeal bread.

Corned Beef & Pickle Sandwich

Use 1 dspn pickle to spread over 2 medium slices wholemeal bread. Fill with lean corned beef and tomato slices.

Chicken, Turkey, Ham or Quorn Salad Sandwich

Use 1 tsp low-fat spread to cover 2 medium slices wholemeal bread. Fill with lettuce, tomato, cucumber and lean slices of chicken, turkey, ham or Quorn Deli slices.

Smoked Mackerel Salad

Prepare a large No-Check salad. Add some smoked mackerel fillets (may be topped with black pepper or mustard seeds). Serve with 1 medium slice bread with 1 tsp low-fat spread.

Mini Chicken Fillets Salad

Checks to count 4

Prepare a large No-Check salad. Add plain or flavoured mini chicken fillets (e.g. coriander & lime, tomato & basil, tikka, etc.). Serve with 1 medium slice bread with 1 tsp low-fat spread.

Roast Beef, Coleslaw & New Potato Salad

Checks to count 5

Prepare a large No-Check salad. Roughly chop 4 small cooked new potatoes and mix with 1 rounded tbsp low-calorie coleslaw. Serve together with some lean, cold roast beef (or other lean cooked meat).

Ham & Egg Salad

Checks to count 5

Prepare a large No-Check salad. Add some lean ham, 1 hard-boiled egg and 1 dspn low-calorie mayonnaise. Serve with 1 medium slice bread with 1 tsp low-fat spread.

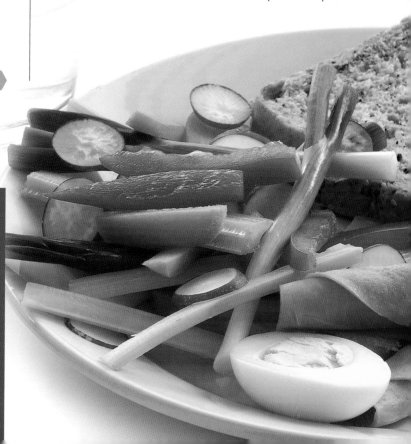

Reminder!

You can make endless different salads – prepare No-Check salad veg, add No-Need-To-Count meat or fish, pulses or vegetarian alternative. Then just add Checks for dressings (unless they are No-Check), pickles or chutney and any breads or spreads.

Sausage Fajita

Checks to count 5

Grill 1 very low fat sausage, then cut into slices. Sauté about 30g sliced onion and 60g sliced red (or other colour) pepper in a pan sprayed with oil until softened. Mix in the sausage slices. Spread mixture down the centre of 1 Discovery Foods Soft Flour Tortilla or Old El Paso Salsa Tortilla. Top with 1 heaped tsp fat-free natural fromage frais, sprinkle with a few drops of Tabasco and roll up.

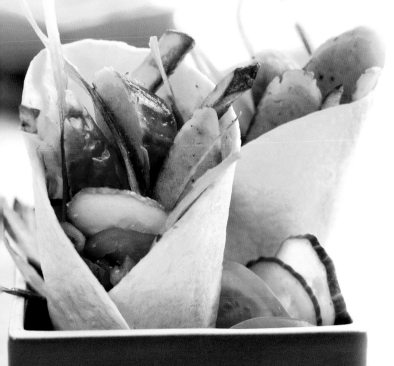

Cottage Cheese Jacket

Checks to count 6

Bake or microwave a 200g potato. Split and fill with cottage cheese (with added pineapple or chive & onion if you prefer). Serve with a large No-Check salad.

Beans & Cheese Choice

Checks to count 6

Warm about 200g baked beans (preferably reduced-sugar-and-salt) and serve over either 2 medium slices toast or a 200g potato, jacket baked or microwaved. Top with a little grated half-fat cheese.

Sardines on Toast

Checks to count 3

Gently warm some sardines in tomato sauce and serve over 1 medium slice wholemeal toast.

Lean Burger

Checks to count 6

Grill either 1 Iceland Good Choice Quarter Pounder or Tesco Healthy Living Quarter Pounder or 2 Quorn Burgers or 2 Linda McCartney Flame Grilled Burgers. Lightly toast 1 burger bap and fill with lettuce, tomato slices and the burger(s). Add 1 Check for a couple of teaspoons pickle or relish.

Lentil & Vegetable Soup

Checks to count 0

Place 30g split red lentils in a saucepan with a small chopped carrot and onion, a small stick of finely sliced celery and a handful of small cauliflower florets. Add 300ml water, bring to the boil, cover and simmer gently 20 minutes. Stir in 1 dspn tomato purée and 1 Oxo vegetable cube or 1 tsp Marigold Vegetable Bouillon and simmer 5 minutes more. Crush vegetables and add extra water if too thick. Add 3 Checks if you wish to eat the soup with 1 medium slice bread.

Broccoli & Cheese Pudding

Checks to count 3

Boil or microwave 100g small broccoli florets. Drain well and place in a small 1 pint ovenproof dish. Crumb 1 medium slice white or wholemeal bread, grate 40g mature half-fat cheddar and mix both with broccoli. Beat 1 egg and make up to 200ml with skimmed milk. Season with black pepper. Pour over broccoli mixture and leave to stand 5 minutes. Bake in a pre-heated oven 190C/gas 5 for 25-30 minutes until golden and firm to the touch. Either eat warm from the bowl, or run a palette knife around the edge and underneath, drain any liquid, turn out, allow to cool and refrigerate to eat cold cut into wedges with some No-Check salad.

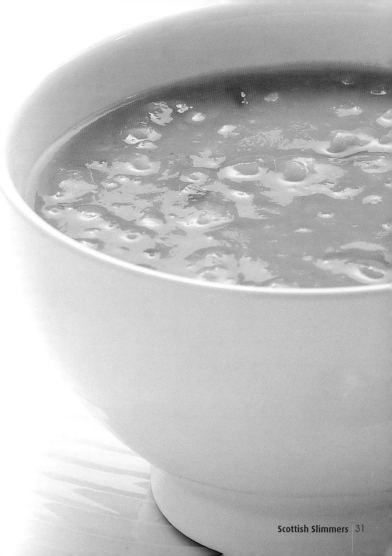

Main Meals

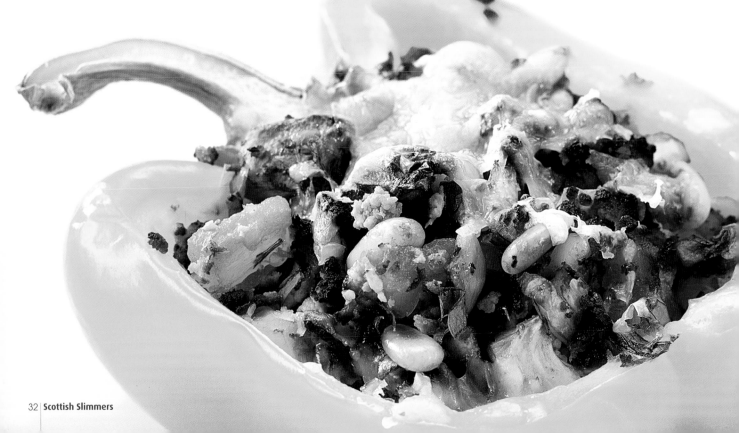

Stuffed Peppers

Boil 45g rice. Brown 100g lean beef, pork or Quorn mince, a small chopped onion and 1 clove crushed garlic in a non-stick pan. Cover and cook gently 5 minutes. Stir in 1 tbsp Oxo gravy granules, 1 tbsp tomato purée, ½ tsp mixed herbs and the cooked rice. Cut a large red or green pepper in half to make 2 shells and remove seeds. Fill with mince mixture, place in a covered dish with 1 tbsp water and microwave on high 4 minutes, or until pepper is tender, or bake 20-30 minutes in a moderate oven. Serve with No-Check vegetables.

Roast Dinner

Serve a medium portion of any lean roast meat or Quorn Chicken Style Roast with gravy made from 1 dspn Oxo or Bisto Best gravy granules and 75ml boiling water. Boil 175g potato, then cut into 2-3 chunks, or drain 300g can new potatoes. Spray with oil and roast 20-30 minutes (whilst cooking meat). Serve with No-Check vegetables. Add 2 Checks for a mini frozen Yorkshire pudding or rounded tbsp of stuffing.

Mince & Tatties

Boil 175g potato with some carrot or swede/turnip. Brown a medium portion of lean mince with chopped onion, carrot and celery (optional). Cover and cook very gently 10 minutes, stirring occasionally. Pour over gravy made from 1 dspn Oxo or Bisto Best gravy granules and 150ml boiling water and simmer 5-10 minutes more. Mash potato and carrot/swede with a little skimmed milk. Serve with green No-Check vegetables. If preferred, mince can be transferred to a suitable dish, topped with potato mixture and browned under a hot grill.

Cheese & Tomato Omelette

Spray a non-stick pan with oil and heat. Pour in 2 beaten eggs and some chopped tomato. When set underneath sprinkle over 30-40g mature grated half-fat cheddar and place under the grill until cheese has melted. Serve with baked beans, preferably reduced-sugar-and salt, and/or No-Check salad. Add 4 Checks for 1 medium slice bread and 1 tsp low-fat spread.

Reminder!

Choose a variety of meals each week to help ensure you get the range of nutrients needed for good health.

Fruity Gammon

Checks to count 6

Boil or microwave 175g potato, then cut into wedges. Spray with oil and brown under the grill. Grill a well trimmed gammon steak with 1 pineapple ring or a canned-in-juice drained peach half. Serve with No-Check vegetables.

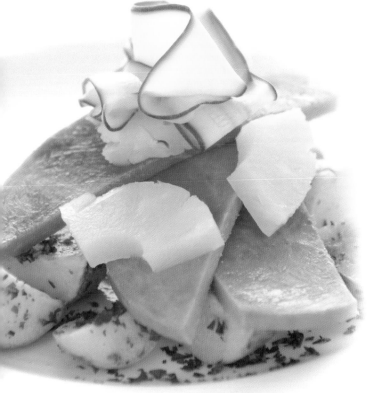

Reminder!

There's no need to count sweetcorn and frozen peas on this plan.

Steak & Jacket

Checks to count 6

Grill a lean medium steak to your liking. Microwave or ovenbake a 200g potato in it's jacket and top with some virtually-fat-free natural yoghurt or fromage frais and chopped chives. Serve with No-Check salad or vegetables.

Lamb/Pork Chops & New Potatoes

Checks to count 5

Grill well trimmed lamb chops or pork chop. Serve with gravy made from 1 dspn Oxo or Bisto Best gravy granules and 75ml boiling water, 150g new potatoes and No-Check vegetables.

Sausage & Mash

Checks to count 6

Grill a couple of very low fat sausages (e.g. Wall's Lean Recipe, or supermarket own brand up to 75 calories each, or Quorn). Boil 175g potato and mash with a little skimmed milk. Slice 1 onion and cook in pan sprayed with oil. Make gravy from 1 dspn Oxo or Bisto Best gravy granules and 75ml boiling water, mix with onions and pour over sausages. Serve with carrots and cabbage or other No-Check vegetables.

Fish in Sauce

 Checks to count 6

Boil/microwave an individual portion of fish in butter or parsley sauce. Serve over boiled rice made from 45g dry weight, accompanied by broccoli or other No-Check vegetables.

Salmon or Trout

 Checks to count 5

Steam, microwave, grill, or pan-fry in spray oil a medium portion of salmon or trout. Serve with 175g new potatoes and No-Check vegetables.

Smoked Salmon & Courgette Tagliatelle

Checks to count 8

Spray a pan with oil and heat. Cover the base with some sliced courgette and allow to brown. Turn slices over and brown other side. Meanwhile, boil 60g dried or 75g fresh tagliatelle, then drain in a colander. In the same saucepan put 50g light soft cheese and 3 tbsp skimmed milk. Heat very gently, stirring until melted. Add extra milk if too thick. Stir in drained pasta until coated. Mix with cooked courgettes and about 75g smoked salmon trimmings. Season well with black pepper.

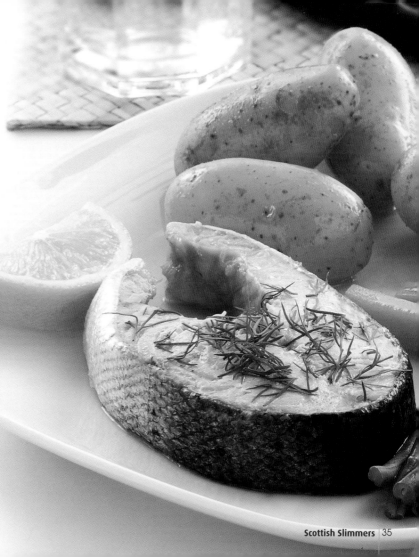

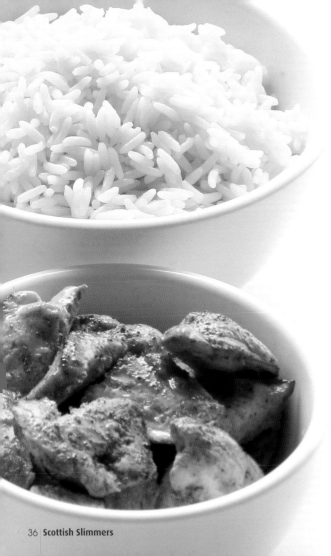

Lemon & Rosemary Chicken

Checks to count: 6

Place a chicken breast on a square of foil, season to taste, top with 2 slices lemon and a sprig of rosemary and wrap into a parcel. Place parcel on a baking tray and cook in a pre-heated oven 190C/gas 5 approximately 25 minutes. Serve with 175g potatoes, gravy made from 1 dspn Oxo or Bisto Best gravy granules and 75ml boiling water, and No-Check vegetables.

Chicken/Quorn Tikka/Tandoori

Checks to count: 6

Cut 1 medium skinless chicken breast into cubes or use a medium portion of Quorn pieces. Marinate 30 minutes in half a 150g pot virtually-fat-free natural yoghurt mixed with 1 dspn tikka or tandoori powder. Remove chicken. Cook in hot oven or under grill 15 minutes. Make dip from remaining half-pot of yoghurt by adding a pinch of mint or ½ tsp mint sauce and grated cucumber (optional). Serve with a large No-Check salad and either 1 mini naan (up to 150 calories) or 1 pitta bread or 45g dry weight boiled rice.

Ham & Cheese Filled Chicken

Checks to count: 6

Wrap 1 slice thin ham around 15g half-fat cheddar. Slit a pocket in a skinless chicken breast and push in ham-wrapped cheese. Secure with a wooden cocktail stick. Cook chicken in pan sprayed with oil approximately 25 minutes, turning halfway through. Serve with 175g potatoes boiled and mashed with a little skimmed milk, gravy made from 1 dspn Oxo or Bisto Best gravy granules and 75ml boiling water, and No-Check vegetables.

Saucy Supper

Checks to count 8

Take a medium portion of any No-Need-To-Count meat, poultry, fish or vegetarian alternative and cook according to instructions in 125g (quarter of a 500g jar) any low-fat "healthy" cooking sauce that has up to 80 calories per 100g. Serve with either 150g potatoes or 30g dry weight pasta, rice, couscous or noodles. Add No-Check vegetables. You can deduct 1 Check if sauce has 60 or less calories per 100g!

Stroganoff

Checks to count 6

Take a medium portion of pork fillet, lean steak, chicken, turkey or Quorn pieces and cut into thin slices or strips appropriately. Brown in pan sprayed with oil. Remove. Add sliced onion, crushed garlic, 2-3 sliced mushrooms, 2 tbsp water, 1 tsp tomato purée and seasoning to taste. Cover and sweat gently 10 minutes stirring occasionally. Return meat to pan and heat. Remove pan from heat and stir in 2 rounded tbsp virtually-fat-free natural fromage frais. Warm gently 30 seconds, stirring. Serve with 45g dry weight, boiled rice or tagliatelle and No-Check vegetables.

Sausage Casserole

Checks to count 6

Put sliced carrot, onion and celery into a saucepan with 200g canned tomatoes and half an Oxo chicken cube. Bring to the boil, cover and simmer until vegetables are tender. Stir occasionally and add a little water if necessary. Grill 2 very low-fat sausages (e.g. Wall's Lean Recipe, Quorn) then cut into chunks. Add sausages to vegetables and simmer 5-10 minutes. Serve with 200g potato boiled and mashed with a little skimmed milk.

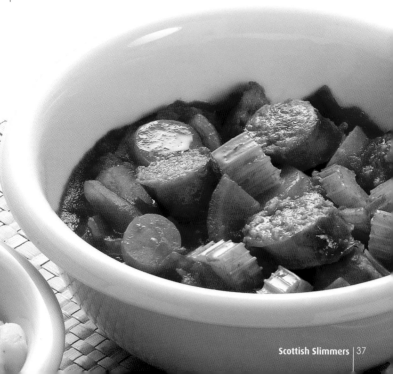

Chicken Aloo Saag

Checks to count 8

Soften 1 sliced onion in a saucepan sprayed with oil. Add 1 cubed chicken breast and stir-fry 3-4 minutes. Add 1 level tbsp Patak's Korma curry paste and 175g potato, peeled and cut into small cubes. Stir-fry 1 minute. Add 200g canned tomatoes and 2 chunks of frozen spinach. Bring to the boil and stir to break up spinach. Turn down heat, cover and simmer gently about 20 minutes until potato is cooked.

Middle Eastern Lamb with Couscous

Checks to count 8

Cook 1 small chopped onion in spray oil until soft. Cut a medium portion lean lamb into cubes and add to the pan. Stir-fry a few minutes until cooked through. Add a pinch of cinnamon and cumin and 1 tsp turmeric and allow to warm a few seconds. Stir in 150ml stock and 4 ready-to-eat apricots. Bring to the boil, cover and simmer 2-3 minutes. Turn off heat and stir in 45g couscous. Re-cover and leave 2-3 minutes for couscous to swell and absorb juices. Fluff up with a fork before serving with oven-roasted peppers and courgettes or other No-Check vegetables.

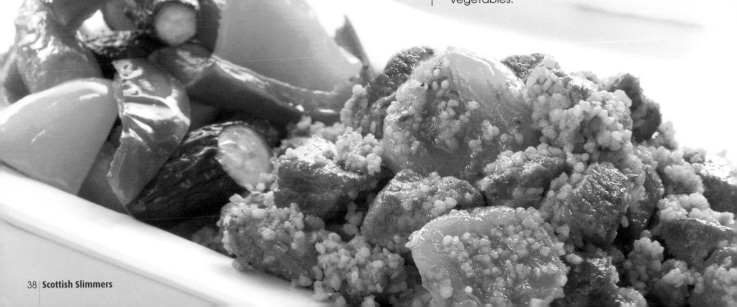

Pasta Bolognese

Brown a medium portion of lean mince in a non-stick pan together with a small chopped onion and garlic to taste. Add 200g canned tomatoes, 1 dspn tomato purée, half an Oxo cube and a pinch of Italian seasoning or mixed herbs. If you wish, add some chopped mushrooms and peppers. Stir well and simmer until sauce thickens. Boil 60g dried or 75g fresh pasta and serve topped with sauce and a little grated half-fat cheese.

Steak, Mangetout & Baby Sweetcorn Stir-fry

Cut a medium portion of lean rump steak into narrow strips and marinate 30 minutes in a mixture of 1 dspn dark soy sauce, 1 dspn sherry and good pinch of ground ginger. Spray pan with oil, heat then brown the steak 2-3 minutes. Add 6 fresh or frozen mangetout or a few sliced green beans, 6 fresh or canned baby sweetcorn, 2 sliced spring onions, 2-3 roughly chopped mushrooms and any remaining marinade. Stir-fry 2-3 minutes. Serve with 45g dry weight, boiled rice or noodles.

Ready Meal

If you wish to have a "healthy" ready meal that includes rice or pasta or potatoes, for this plan only, you can assume that these will account for approximately half the calories of the meal. Therefore, if a meal has

approximately 400 calories   **Checks to count** 8

approximately 350 calories   **Checks to count** 7

approximately 300 calories   **Checks to count** 6

Chilli Tacos/Rice

Brown a medium portion of lean mince with 1 small chopped onion and garlic to taste. Add 200g canned tomatoes, 1 dspn tomato purée, some sliced peppers, 2-3 tbsp canned kidney beans, a pinch of cumin and 1 tsp chilli powder, or to taste. Simmer until vegetables are tender. Season to taste. Serve mixture in 3 taco shells topped with a little grated half-fat cheese accompanied by a No-Check salad. If preferred, omit taco shells and serve with 45g dry weight, boiled rice.

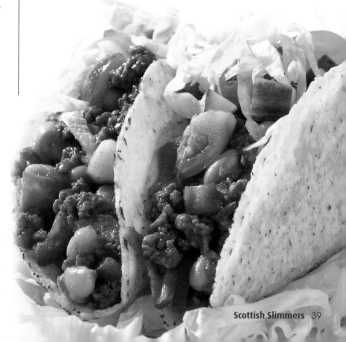

Ten Ways
When Socialising

①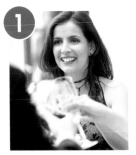

On this plan there's no need to "save" Checks for socialising or meals out. Don't forget you have a Special Weekly Allowance of 20 extra Checks which can be used for this purpose. You don't have to use these Checks if you don't need them.

②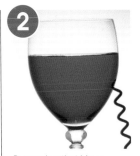

Remember that binge drinking is not good for health, nor your waistline! See Socialising Check Lists on page 45 for what you'll need to count.

③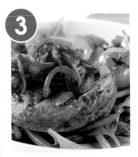

On this plan there's no need to count Checks in plain grilled meats and fish provided they are not smothered in a rich creamy or buttery or cheesy sauce. Lean roast meats are another alternative. You will need to add Checks for any bread, potatoes, pasta or rice you have. See Socialising Check Lists on page 45.

④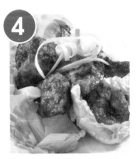

Tandoori or tikka (without the masala sauce) chicken or prawns are the best choices in an Indian restaurant (No-Need-To-Count on this plan). Next best choices are Chicken Jalfrezi or Chicken Rogan Josh or a Chicken, Prawn or Vegetable Balti (also No-Need-To-Count on this plan).

⑤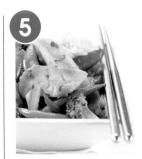

In a Chinese restaurant, avoid battered foods and sweet sauces. Meat, chicken, duck, prawns or tofu stir-fried with vegetables (e.g. with mushroom, pepper or spring onion) or in a blackbean or oyster sauce are No-Need-To-Count on this plan.

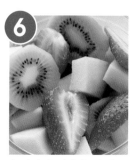

6

A saintly fresh fruit salad is ideal for dessert. Count around 4 Checks, or nothing if you have it as your 2 average Every Day Bonus servings of fruit.

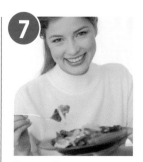

7

If you really have no idea how to count your meal out, have moderate portions of what takes your fancy and assume you will have spent your 20 Special Weekly Allowance Checks!

8

If you are familiar with the restaurant's menu, plan in advance what you intend to have and avoid looking at the menu so you are not tempted to change your mind.

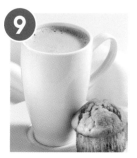

9

Remember that on this plan, skimmed milk is a No-Need-To-Count food, so provided it's a "skinny" latte (made with skimmed milk), you don't need to count it. The same goes for a "skinny" cappuccino, but count 1 Check if you have the chocolate topping!

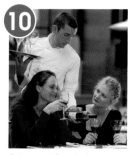

10

Enjoy your food but remember that the prime purpose of socialising is to enjoy the company of friends and family.

Check Lists

These are the Checks you need to count on this plan. (Some may be different from usual Positive Eating values.)

Energy Foods

1 small slice bread	2
1 medium slice bread	3
1 thick slice bread	4
50g bread roll	5
60g pitta bread	6
40g tortilla or wrap	5

30g breakfast cereal, average	4
45g breakfast cereal, average	6
2 Weetabix	5
2 Shredded Wheat	6

150g potatoes	4
175g potatoes	5
200g potatoes	6
300g potatoes	8
100g frozen-weight low-fat oven chips	5
100g baked-weight low-fat oven chips	7

Pasta, rice, noodles, couscous, bulghur:

30g dry/75g boiled	4
45g dry/115g boiled	6
60g dry/150g boiled	8

1 taco shell	2
1 mini frozen Yorkshire pudding	2
1 large frozen Yorkshire pudding	4

1 medium parsnip	2
100g sweet potato or yams	4

Miscellaneous Products

1 fish finger, grilled	1
1 fish cake, grilled	2
100g portion battered/breaded fish, ovenbaked	8
1 breaded chicken portion, ovenbaked	8
1 breaded Quorn portion, ovenbaked	4

Cheese & Dairy

Remember, on this plan, there's no need to count skimmed milk, half-fat (or less) cheeses or virtually-fat-free yoghurt and fromage frais!

30g Cheddar or Cheshire	5
30g Brie or Camembert	4
30g Edam or Feta	4
1 dspn grated Parmesan	1
150ml semi-skimmed or soya milk	1

Bits & Pieces

1 tsp low-fat spread	1
1 tsp butter or oil	1.5
1 rounded tbsp half-fat crème fraiche	2
1 tbsp apple sauce	1
2 dspn brown sauce or tomato ketchup	1
1 tbsp pickles or chutney	1
2 dspn low-calorie salad cream	1
1 dspn low-calorie mayonnaise	1
1 dspn Bisto Best or Oxo gravy granules	1
1 dspn cornflour	1
1 tbsp Patak's Korma or Madras Curry Paste	3
1 tbsp Patak's Tandoori or Tikka Curry Paste	1
1 tsp chopped nuts or sesame seeds	1
1 tsp pine kernels	1
5 olives	1
2 tbsp wine	1
1 tbsp sherry	1
75ml/5 tbsp passata	1
75ml/5 tbsp low-fat pasta sauce	1
1 tsp sugar or honey or syrup	1
1 tsp jam, marmalade or lemon curd	1
2 tsp reduced-sugar jam or marmalade	1
1 tsp peanut butter	2
1 rounded tbsp raisins or sultanas	2
2 ready-to-eat apricots	1
1 date or small dried fig	1
3 prunes	2

Savoury Snacks

1 Paterson's Oatcake	2
1 Ryvita Original or Dark Rye	1
1 Ryvita Multigrain or Sunflower & Oats	1.5
1 Ryvita Pumpkin & Oats	2
2 cream crackers	2.5
1 rice cake	1
1 large or 2 small water biscuits	1
25g Jacob's Thai Bites	4
28g Kellogg's Special K Lite Bites	5
30g Quaker Crispy Snack-a-Jacks, average	5
25g Twiglets Original	4
20g Boots Shapers Crinkle Crisps	4
24g Boots Shapers Manhattan Style Pretzels	3
Marks & Spencer Count On Us snacks, average	4
25g Popping corn, microwaved without fat	4
10-15g Sainsbury's BGTY Fries, Bacon Waffles, Onion Rings	2
19g Walkers French Fries	4
23g Walkers Potato Heads	4
25g Walkers Square Crisps	4
25g Almonds, cashews, hazelnuts, pistachios	6
25g Brazil nuts, pecans, walnuts	7
25g Peanuts	6
25g Nuts & raisins	4
25g Pumpkin seeds or sunflower seeds	6

Sweet Treats

Fox's Officially Low Fat Minis 40g	6
Go Ahead! Cookie	3
Go Ahead! Yoghurt Break, 2 slice pack	5
McVitie's Light Digestive or Light Hob Nob	2.5
McVitie's Light Milk Chocolate Digestive	3
McVitie's Light Rich Tea	1.5
Scottish Slimmers Mini Cookies 26g pack	5

Jordans Frusli	5
Jordans Honey & Almond Crunchy Bar	5
Kellogg's Nutri-grain Bar	5
Kellogg's Special K Bar	4
M&S Count On Us Cereal Bar	3
Nestlé Fitnesse or Sveltesse Bar	4
Quaker Chewee Bar	4
Quaker Dipps	5

Asda Good For You! Cake Slice, av.	3
Cadbury's Milk Chocolate Mini Roll	5
Go Ahead! Choc Chip Cake Bar	4
Go Ahead! Crispy Flapjack	4
Mr Kipling Angel Slice or Country Slice	5
Mr Kipling Victoria Slice	4
Mr Kipling French Fancy	4
Tesco Healthy Living Cake Slice, av.	3
Tunnock's Tea Cake	4

Cadbury's Curly Wurly	5
Cadbury's Dairy Milk 17.5g	4
Chupa Chups Cremosa Sugar Free Lolly	1
Mars Fun Size 20g	4
Milky Way 26g	5
Nestlé 2-finger Kit Kat	4
Sula Sugar Free Sweets, 50g box	5
Trebor Sugar Free Mints, mini box	3

1 meringue nest	2
100g supermarket own-brand crème caramel	4
Ambrosia Low Fat Devon Custard 150g	4
Cadbury's Light Mousse 55g	3
Danone Shape Fruit Juice Mousse	5
M&S Count On Us Choc & Caramel Dream 130g	5
M&S Count On Us Choc & Cherry Dessert 115g	5
Muller 99% Fat Free Rice 150g	5
Sainsbury BGTY Blackcurrant Fool 113g	4
Sainsbury BGTY Strawberry Trifle 125g	5

60ml level scoop plain ice cream	2
Iceland Good Choice Chocolate & Vanilla Lolly	2.5
Mackie's Vibrant Low Fat Sorbet, 60ml scoop	2
Nestlé Orange Maid	2
Skinny Cow Very Berry Stick	3
Skinny Cow Cookies & Cream Stick	4
Tesco Fruit Swirl or Heavenly Swirl	4
Wall's Mini Milk	1

Check Lists for Socialising

Drinks

1 small glass wine	4
25ml single shot of any spirit	2
35ml shot of any spirit	3
275-330ml/half pint average beer, lager, or cider	4
275ml bottle "alcopop"	8
275ml Bacardi Breezer Half Sugar	5
275ml Archers Vea	5

The following can be used for typical servings:

Bread stick	1
Dinner roll	5
Butter pat	3
Poppadum	3
Naan bread	15
Jacket potato, medium	8
New potatoes	6
Roast potatoes, 3 chunks	9
Main course pasta	14
Takeaway portion of boiled noodles	12
Takeaway portion of fried noodles	16
Boiled rice, per rounded serving spoon	2
Fried or pilau rice, per rounded serving spoon	3

Main Courses

There's no need to count the following :

Any lean roast meat with a little gravy
Grilled steak
Grilled gammon (fat removed)
Any lean grilled meat with fat removed
Any grilled or steamed fish

The above may be served with a tomato-based sauce but avoid cream, butter or cheese sauces.

Chicken Tikka or Tandoori (no masala sauce)
Chicken, prawn or vegetable Balti
Chicken, prawn or vegetable Jalfrezi
Chicken, prawn or vegetable Rogan Josh

Stir-fried beef, chicken, duck, pork, prawns with vegetables, or in blackbean or oyster sauce.

Desserts

Fresh fruit salad	4
2 round scoops ice cream or sorbet	8
Pies or flans or gateau or 4 profiteroles	16
Topping of cream or serving of custard	4

Ten Ways to
Increase Your Activity

1

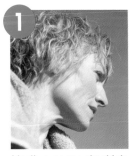

Ideally everyone should do 30 minutes of moderate-intensity activity on most days. If you never seem to have half an hour to spare, break it down into three 10-minute spurts.

2

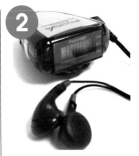

Start wearing a pedometer to count how many steps you do each day. We should all be aiming for 10,000 a day, but don't worry if you are nowhere near this to start off with. Use the pedometer to see if you can do a few more steps each day.

3

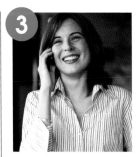

Walk as you talk on your mobile or cordless phone. A half-hour call can easily clock up 2,000 steps!

4

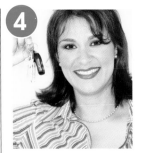

Think about how you could use the car less often – and act on your thoughts.

5

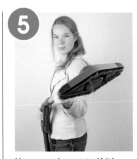

Housework counts if it's done with vim and vigour – you'll finish your chores much more quickly too!

6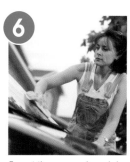

Forget the car wash and do it yourself.

7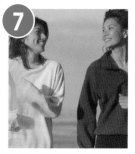

Find a buddy and commit to doing an hour of something active together every week.

8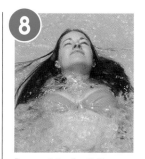

Do a variety of activities – sometimes walk, sometimes cycle, sometimes swim, sometimes dance. Anything that takes your fancy. Everything to prevent boredom.

9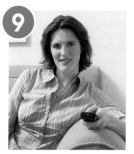

Watch less television. Makes sense, doesn't it?

10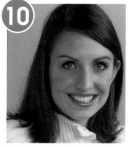

Always bear in mind that there's more to being active than just burning extra calories – as if that wasn't good enough! If you are active on a daily basis, your metabolism revs up and tends to stay revved up so you continue to burn extra calories even when the activity has stopped. How good is that for weight management!

What if...

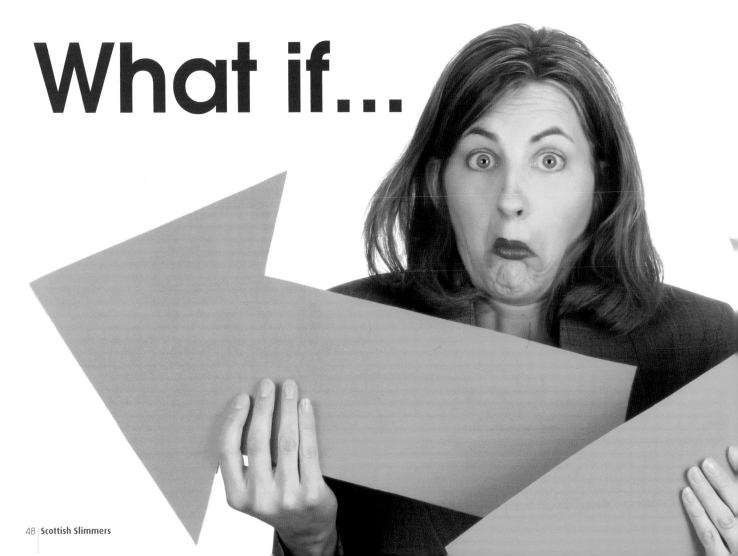

What if I want to eat a No-Need-To-Count food between meals?

If you have spent all your Checks for the day, and eaten your Every Day Bonus fruit, milk/yoghurt and had plenty of No-Check veggies but are still hungry, it's unlikely to slow down your weight loss if you have a small amount of a No-Need-To-Count food such as a little ham or small piece of half-fat cheese to keep you going between meals.

What if I want to eat something that's not on this plan?

Most Essential Extras, such as alcohol, biscuits, cakes, crisps, desserts, have the same Check value as on the normal PEP (Positive Eating Plan). Many of the better choices are included in the Check Lists in this book, but you can also use your Check Book for these types of foods.

Breads, cereals, potatoes, pasta, rice, bulghur, couscous, noodles, etc. are also counted as on the normal PEP, and so are sauces, gravies and other bits and pieces you might want to add to a meal. Remember, though that there are many No-Check ways to flavour food (see Every Day Bonus Free Additions on page 11).

In the Check Lists, under Miscellaneous Products, you will find the values for some breaded or battered products. The values are different from the PEP as they include both No-Need-To-Count items and things that should be counted. See page 39 if you want to know how to count a "healthy" ready meal.

This plan doesn't have quite as much variety and flexibility as the full PEP – but the trade-off is that there are many more foods that you don't have to count at all!

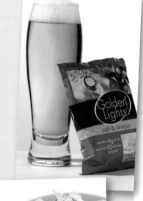

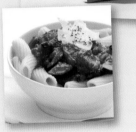

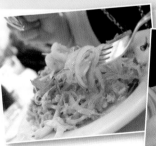

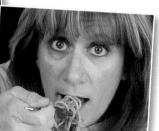

What if I go over my daily Checks allowance?

If it's just a Check or two, you could try and cut back by the same amount the next day. If it's considerably more, take it out of your Special Weekly Allowance of 20 Checks.

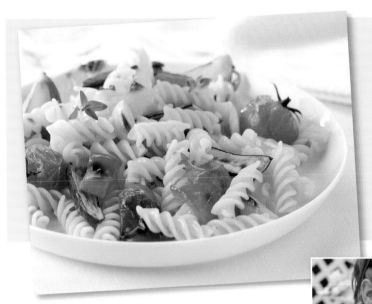

What if I don't use all my daily Checks allowance?

It doesn't matter if you don't use up every Check, every day, but don't starve yourself! Eating too little on a regular basis can slow down your weight loss as your metabolism will wind down in order to try and conserve energy.

You should be spending most of your Checks on energy-providing foods such as breads, cereals, potatoes, rice and pasta which will also boost your fibre intake, especially if you choose wholegrain or wholemeal varieties.

It's best not to carry over any unused Checks to the next day. You don't have to consciously "save" Checks on this plan as you have your Special Weekly Allowance, should you need it.

What if I don't use all or any of my Special Weekly Allowance?

It doesn't matter, but don't carry over any unused Checks to the next week. Start each week with a new Special Weekly Allowance.

What if I want to use a meal from the PEP?

For simplicity, treat it as though it was a "healthy" ready meal and count just half the Checks. (See page 39).

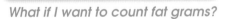

What if I want to count fat grams?

Most Every Day Bonus foods and No-Need-To-Count foods are low in fat and, as you only have 20 Checks a day to spend on other foods (or 30 if you are a man), it would be hard to eat too much fat on this plan provided you stick by the rules. Therefore, there's no need to count fat on this plan.

What if I start on this plan but during the day need to change over to using the PEP?

Write down all you have eaten so far (except No-Check foods) and count the Checks for these – as you would normally do when using the PEP. Take this number away from your normal PEP daily allowance of Checks, then take off another 3 Checks, and that's how many Checks you have left to spend. You can still use Checks from your Special Weekly Allowance if you need them. (As you won't have weighed No-Need-To-Count foods, you may have to estimate how much you have had.)

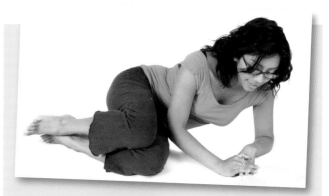

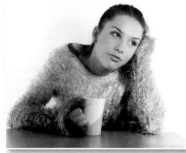

Are you really trying to be a little more active?

Remember that everyone loses weight at a different rate. Lighter people, or those who are near target weight will tend to lose less than heavier people or those who have only recently started a weight loss plan.

What if I am losing less than 2lb a week?

Check you are not having too many or too large portions of No-Need-To-Count foods.

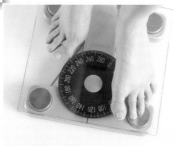

What if I want to use the PEP on some days and this plan on others?

It's probably best not to keep chopping and changing from one day to the next, but if, for example, you have a social occasion to attend and think this plan might not be flexible enough for you, start the whole day using the PEP and count your normal daily allowance of Checks – less 3 Checks! (The 3 missing Checks are really that day's contribution to your Special Weekly Allowance.) This means you can still use Checks from your Special Weekly Allowance also, if you need them. Before you decide to go this route, take a look at the "Check List for Socialising" on page 45. You may decide you could stay on this plan even though you are socialising.

Remember, if you switch to the PEP, there aren't any No-Need-To-Count foods! (other than normal No-Check foods).

Ten Ways of Coping

①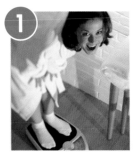

Set small achievable goals.

②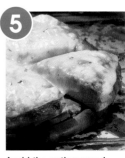

Accept you won't be perfect – but there's no harm in trying!

③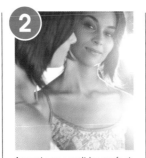

Food doesn't have a brain – it can't solve your problems. Get support from friends, family or neutral counsellors. Bear in mind that ordinary people are not mind readers – you need to ask for their help. You can return the favour when they are at a low ebb.

④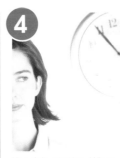

Use delay tactics. When the urge to eat strikes even though you know you are not hungry, wait 10 minutes. Turn your attention to something else and very often the urge passes.

⑤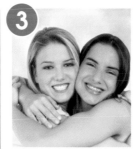

Avoid the eating round syndrome. If you simply must have a specific food and nothing else will do, don't waste Checks on foods you really don't want. Have the desired item, count it and forget it.

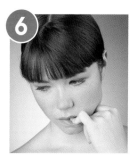

Don't worry about things over which you have no control.

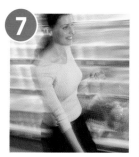

Don't set yourself up to fail. Avoidance is sometimes the best policy. Avoid having your "can't resist foods" in the house. Avoid walking past bakers, coffee shops or chip shops – the aromas are meant to tempt you!

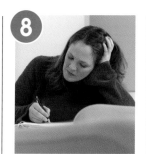

Get organised – write out "to do" lists, plan your shopping and start to de-junk. You'll feel so much more in control.

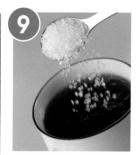

You have to practise good habits until they are more natural than the bad habits they replace, but don't try and change everything at once. Make a small change to start with – for example, half a teaspoon less sugar in your tea – and go with it until you feel comfortable with it. Then move on to the next challenge.

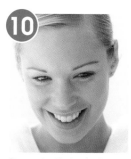

Recognise that nobody is good at everything but most people are good at something – you included! Give yourself credit for those things you do well.

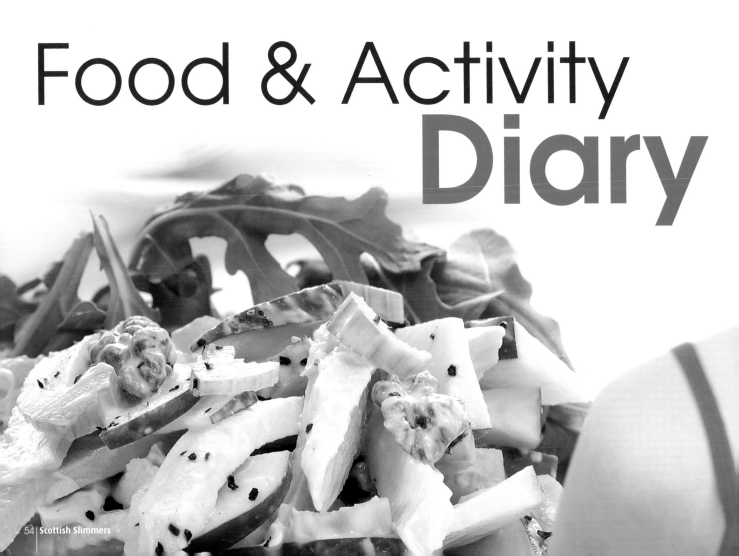

Food & Activity Diary

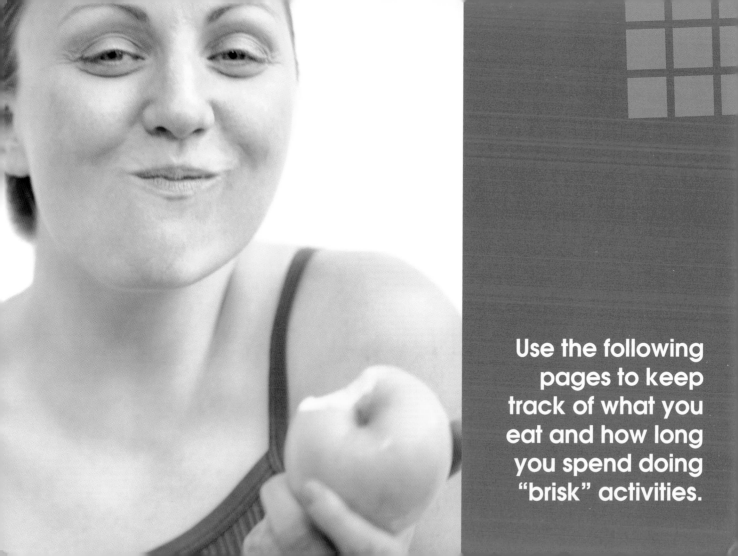

Use the following pages to keep track of what you eat and how long you spend doing "brisk" activities.

Week 1

Date:	Checks	Date:	Checks	Date:	Checks	Date:	Checks

Total Checks today:		Total Checks today:		Total Checks today:		Total Checks today:	
Every Day Bonus:		**Every Day Bonus:**		**Every Day Bonus:**		**Every Day Bonus:**	
1 bone-builder	◯	1 bone-builder	◯	1 bone-builder	◯	1 bone-builder	◯
2 fruits	◯◯	2 fruits	◯◯	2 fruits	◯◯	2 fruits	◯◯
3 veg (at least)	◯◯◯	3 veg (at least)	◯◯◯	3 veg (at least)	◯◯◯	3 veg (at least)	◯◯◯
8 drinks	◯◯◯◯◯◯◯◯	8 drinks	◯◯◯◯◯◯◯◯	8 drinks	◯◯◯◯◯◯◯◯	8 drinks	◯◯◯◯◯◯◯◯

Date:	Checks	Date:	Checks	Date:	Checks	Activities	Minutes
						Monday	
						Tuesday	
						Wednesday	
						Thursday	
						Friday	
						Saturday	
						Sunday	

Total Checks today:	Total Checks today:	Total Checks today:

Every Day Bonus:		Every Day Bonus:		Every Day Bonus:	
1 bone-builder	◯	1 bone-builder	◯	1 bone-builder	◯
2 fruits	◯◯	2 fruits	◯◯	2 fruits	◯◯
3 veg (at least)	◯◯◯	3 veg (at least)	◯◯◯	3 veg (at least)	◯◯◯
8 drinks	◯◯◯◯◯◯◯◯	8 drinks	◯◯◯◯◯◯◯◯	8 drinks	◯◯◯◯◯◯◯◯

Special Weekly Allowance

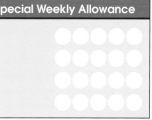

Week 2

Date:	Checks	Date:	Checks	Date:	Checks	Date:	Checks

Total Checks today:		Total Checks today:		Total Checks today:		Total Checks today:	

Every Day Bonus:		Every Day Bonus:		Every Day Bonus:		Every Day Bonus:	
1 bone-builder	○	1 bone-builder	○	1 bone-builder	○	1 bone-builder	○
2 fruits	○○	2 fruits	○○	2 fruits	○○	2 fruits	○○
3 veg (at least)	○○○	3 veg (at least)	○○○	3 veg (at least)	○○○	3 veg (at least)	○○○
8 drinks	○○○○○○○○	8 drinks	○○○○○○○○	8 drinks	○○○○○○○○	8 drinks	○○○○○○○○

Date:	Checks	Date:	Checks	Date:	Checks	Activities	Minutes
						Monday	
						Tuesday	
						Wednesday	
						Thursday	
						Friday	
						Saturday	
						Sunday	

Total Checks today:		**Total Checks today:**		**Total Checks today:**	

Every Day Bonus:		**Every Day Bonus:**		**Every Day Bonus:**	
1 bone-builder	●	1 bone-builder	●	1 bone-builder	●
2 fruits	●●	2 fruits	●●	2 fruits	●●
3 veg (at least)	●●●	3 veg (at least)	●●●	3 veg (at least)	●●●
8 drinks	●●●●●●●●	8 drinks	●●●●●●●●	8 drinks	●●●●●●●●

Special Weekly Allowance

Week 3

Date:	Checks	Date:	Checks	Date:	Checks	Date:	Checks

Total Checks today:		Total Checks today:		Total Checks today:		Total Checks today:	
Every Day Bonus:		**Every Day Bonus:**		**Every Day Bonus:**		**Every Day Bonus:**	
1 bone-builder	⚪	1 bone-builder	⚪	1 bone-builder	⚪	1 bone-builder	⚪
2 fruits	⚪⚪	2 fruits	⚪⚪	2 fruits	⚪⚪	2 fruits	⚪⚪
3 veg (at least)	⚪⚪⚪	3 veg (at least)	⚪⚪⚪	3 veg (at least)	⚪⚪⚪	3 veg (at least)	⚪⚪⚪
8 drinks	⚪⚪⚪⚪⚪⚪⚪⚪	8 drinks	⚪⚪⚪⚪⚪⚪⚪⚪	8 drinks	⚪⚪⚪⚪⚪⚪⚪⚪	8 drinks	⚪⚪⚪⚪⚪⚪⚪⚪

Date:	Checks	Date:	Checks	Date:	Checks

Activities	Minutes
Monday	
Tuesday	
Wednesday	
Thursday	
Friday	
Saturday	
Sunday	

Total Checks today:		Total Checks today:		Total Checks today:	
Every Day Bonus:		**Every Day Bonus:**		**Every Day Bonus:**	
1 bone-builder		1 bone-builder		1 bone-builder	
2 fruits		2 fruits		2 fruits	
3 veg (at least)		3 veg (at least)		3 veg (at least)	
8 drinks		8 drinks		8 drinks	

Special Weekly Allowance

Week 4

Date:	Checks	Date:	Checks	Date:	Checks	Date:	Checks
Total Checks today:		**Total Checks today:**		**Total Checks today:**		**Total Checks today:**	

Every Day Bonus:		Every Day Bonus:		Every Day Bonus:		Every Day Bonus:	
1 bone-builder	○	1 bone-builder	○	1 bone-builder	○	1 bone-builder	○
2 fruits	○○	2 fruits	○○	2 fruits	○○	2 fruits	○○
3 veg (at least)	○○○	3 veg (at least)	○○○	3 veg (at least)	○○○	3 veg (at least)	○○○
8 drinks	○○○○○○○○	8 drinks	○○○○○○○○	8 drinks	○○○○○○○○	8 drinks	○○○○○○○○

Date:	Checks	Date:	Checks	Date:	Checks

Activities	Minutes
Monday	
Tuesday	
Wednesday	
Thursday	
Friday	
Saturday	
Sunday	

Total Checks today:		Total Checks today:		Total Checks today:	
Every Day Bonus:		**Every Day Bonus:**		**Every Day Bonus:**	
1 bone-builder	◯	1 bone-builder	◯	1 bone-builder	◯
2 fruits	◯◯	2 fruits	◯◯	2 fruits	◯◯
3 veg (at least)	◯◯◯	3 veg (at least)	◯◯◯	3 veg (at least)	◯◯◯
8 drinks	◯◯◯◯◯◯◯◯	8 drinks	◯◯◯◯◯◯◯◯	8 drinks	◯◯◯◯◯◯◯◯

Special Weekly Allowance

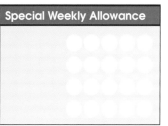

Week 5

Date:	Checks	Date:	Checks	Date:	Checks	Date:	Checks

Total Checks today:		Total Checks today:		Total Checks today:		Total Checks today:	
Every Day Bonus:		**Every Day Bonus:**		**Every Day Bonus:**		**Every Day Bonus:**	
1 bone-builder		1 bone-builder		1 bone-builder		1 bone-builder	
2 fruits		2 fruits		2 fruits		2 fruits	
3 veg (at least)		3 veg (at least)		3 veg (at least)		3 veg (at least)	
8 drinks		8 drinks		8 drinks		8 drinks	

Date:	Checks	Date:	Checks	Date:	Checks	Activities	Minutes
						Monday	
						Tuesday	
						Wednesday	
						Thursday	
						Friday	
						Saturday	
						Sunday	

Total Checks today:		Total Checks today:		Total Checks today:	
Every Day Bonus:		**Every Day Bonus:**		**Every Day Bonus:**	
1 bone-builder	○	1 bone-builder	○	1 bone-builder	○
2 fruits	○○	2 fruits	○○	2 fruits	○○
3 veg (at least)	○○○	3 veg (at least)	○○○	3 veg (at least)	○○○
8 drinks	○○○○○○○○	8 drinks	○○○○○○○○	8 drinks	○○○○○○○○

Special Weekly Allowance

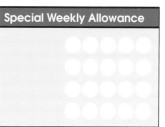

Week 6

Date:	Checks	Date:	Checks	Date:	Checks	Date:	Checks

Total Checks today:		Total Checks today:		Total Checks today:		Total Checks today:	
Every Day Bonus:		Every Day Bonus:		Every Day Bonus:		Every Day Bonus:	
1 bone-builder		1 bone-builder		1 bone-builder		1 bone-builder	
2 fruits		2 fruits		2 fruits		2 fruits	
3 veg (at least)		3 veg (at least)		3 veg (at least)		3 veg (at least)	
8 drinks		8 drinks		8 drinks		8 drinks	

Date:	Checks	Date:	Checks	Date:	Checks	Activities	Minutes
						Monday	
						Tuesday	
						Wednesday	
						Thursday	
						Friday	
						Saturday	
						Sunday	

Total Checks today:		Total Checks today:		Total Checks today:	
Every Day Bonus:		**Every Day Bonus:**		**Every Day Bonus:**	
1 bone-builder	○	1 bone-builder	○	1 bone-builder	○
2 fruits	○○	2 fruits	○○	2 fruits	○○
3 veg (at least)	○○○	3 veg (at least)	○○○	3 veg (at least)	○○○
8 drinks	○○○○○○○○	8 drinks	○○○○○○○○	8 drinks	○○○○○○○○

Special Weekly Allowance

Ten Ways to Stay on Track

1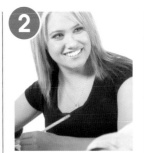

Take into account everything you should count.

2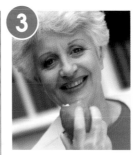

When it comes to weight loss, more people are successful if they keep track of what they eat. Keep filling in the Food & Activity Diary pages.

3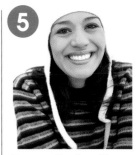

Avoid extreme hunger – always have a piece of fruit handy.

4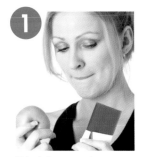

Know when you are most likely to need a snack – for example, in the evening or when preparing the kid's tea – and plan for it.

5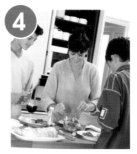

Turn negative thoughts into positive thoughts.

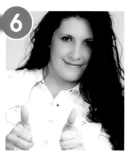

Give your weight loss programme the importance it deserves.

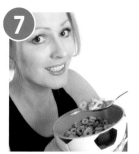

If you eat too much one day, just forget it. You can start again at the next meal or the next day.

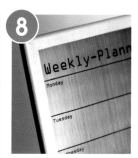

Never wait until Monday.

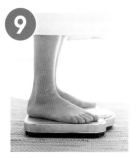

Don't keep hopping on and off the scales or you are sure to be disappointed. Weight normally fluctuates throughout the day. Compare your weekly progress at the same time of day, on the same scales, wearing the same sort of clothing.

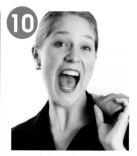

You only have to lose the next pound.

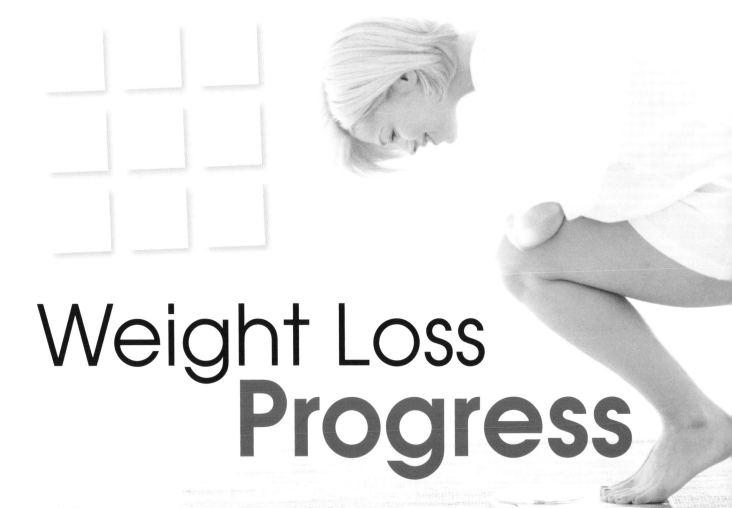

Weight Loss
Progress

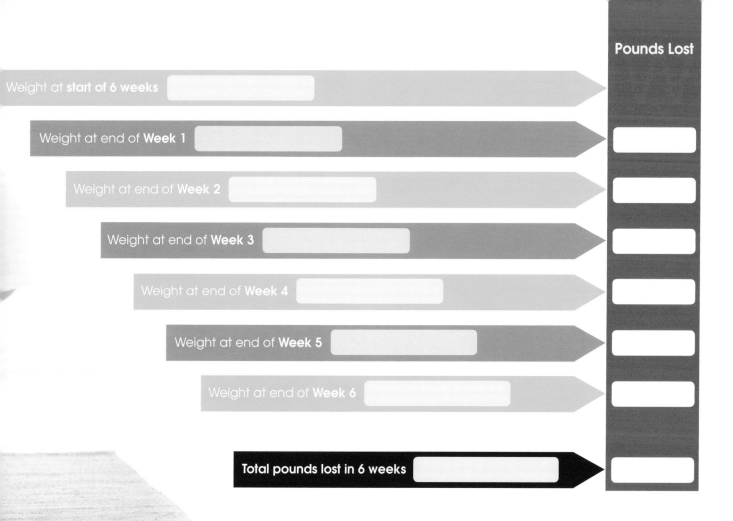

Pounds Lost

Weight at **start of 6 weeks**

Weight at end of **Week 1**

Weight at end of **Week 2**

Weight at end of **Week 3**

Weight at end of **Week 4**

Weight at end of **Week 5**

Weight at end of **Week 6**

Total pounds lost in 6 weeks

What next?

The next stone – and beyond

If you have enjoyed using this plan and wish to continue using it for another six weeks, or even longer, go ahead. You'll know it may not be quite as flexible as the full PEP but, from a nutritional point of view, it doesn't ban any food group and, provided you normally have Every Day Bonus foods and generally choose a wide variety of other foods (another of our favourite "rules"), you will be getting all the nutrition you need.

The choice is really whether or not you prefer the freedom of not having to weigh and count what are essentially low-fat protein foods, e.g. lean meat, fish, pulses and low-fat dairy produce, which comprise "No-Need-To-Count" foods.

Back to the PEP

If, however, you prefer the flexibility of the full PEP, you can go back to using that. Have your usual full daily Check allowance but, don't forget you are lighter now, so check your Positive Eating Plan to ensure you know what your current "usual" daily Check allowance for weight loss should be. It may be a little less than before! Also, don't forget that you will need to spend Checks for all foods except No-Check foods and Every Day Bonus allowances.

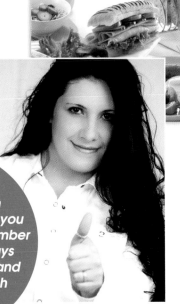

Scottish Slimmers

PEP Complete

Whatever you decide, we wish you all the success you deserve – and remember that you can always count on the help and support of Scottish Slimmers.